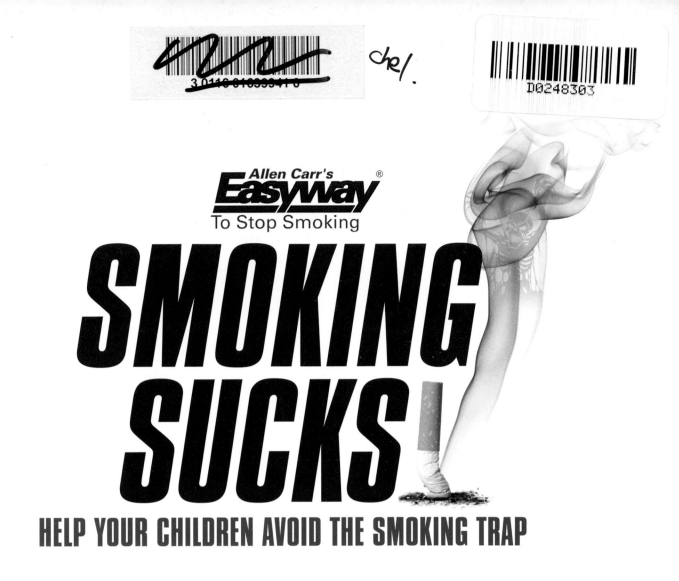

Allen Carr's Easyway®
To Stop Smoking

SMOKING SUCKS!

HELP YOUR CHILDREN AVOID THE SMOKING TRAP

ARCTURUS

ALLEN CARR'S EASYWAY METHOD

Allen Carr's Easyway method has helped over 10 million people to stop smoking throughout the world. *Allen Carr's Easy Way to Stop Smoking* is an internationally bestselling book which has sold over 8 million copies in over 20 different languages, making it easily the most successful book on quitting ever published.

In *Smoking Sucks!* Allen Carr and Robin Hayley, who heads Allen's global organisation, apply the phenomenal success of the Easyway method to the problem of children smoking. They tackle the two main issues: stopping children from starting and encouraging those who are already dabbling to stop. *Smoking Sucks!* is the most effective way of enabling your child to remain, or to become, a happy non-smoker.

Special thanks go to Paul Mason and Steve Beaumont for their amazing writing and illustration skills, to Roberta Bailey, Charles Cooper and Ian McLellan of Arcturus Publishing for helping to make this project happen, and to John Dicey of Allen Carr's Easyway International whose inspiration for conceiving and driving this project forward was drawn from the birth of Emily and Harry Dicey.
Robin Hayley & Allen Carr

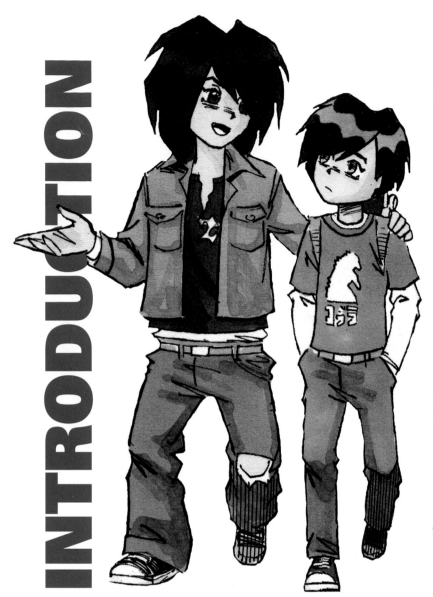

INTRODUCTION

Our children are targets for one of the most ruthless and best-financed marketing machines in the world. Tobacco companies need to target youngsters through marketing and advertising because they need to replace the 110,000 customers their products kill each year in the UK alone. Helping our children to recognize the futility of smoking is the best way we can ensure their health and wellbeing.

THE SMOKING TRAP

Three out of four children are aware of cigarettes before they reach the age of five whether or not their parents smoke. However, studies have found that children whose parents smoke are four times more likely to smoke than children of non-smoking parents. So, if you smoke, your child is already at a terrible disadvantage. You are adding to the efforts of the tobacco industry's marketing machine by being a walking, talking advertisement for smoking. Don't kid yourself; even if they hate the fact that you smoke now, at some stage in their development they will almost certainly see smoking as a rite of passage towards adulthood.

You can rectify that immediately, not for their sake, but for yours. If you don't like the thought of your children smoking, it means that you wish you'd never started

yourself and would rather be a non-smoker. To discover just how easy it can be to quit by using Allen Carr's Easyway method, see the details of our books and clinics at the back of this booklet or at **www.allencarr.com**

Why don't the usual warnings work?
When trying to prevent their children from falling into the smoking trap, parents tend to deliver warnings. Children almost invariably misunderstand these warnings in relation to smoking. They tend to think of warnings from parents as generally falling into one of two categories.

Warning category one:
'Don't do that because I don't approve!'
These are the warnings children are **MOST** likely to ignore. At a certain stage in their development, most

children experience an overwhelming urge to **REBEL**. Examples of these warnings include:

- *'Don't use bad language!'*
- *'Don't play with that friend!'*
- *'Don't stay up late!'*

How many of these sorts of warnings are familiar from your own childhood? How did you react to them? These are the warnings children will almost certainly **IGNORE** at some stage in their life, often as a way of asserting their independence. The consequences of ignoring these warnings are relatively minor, and the children almost certainly know this **BEFORE** they decide to ignore them because of the weak justification given for the warnings:

- *'Don't use bad language because it's rude.'*
- *'Don't play with that friend because I don't like them.'*
- *'Don't stay up late because you'll be tired in the morning.'*

Given the relatively trivial justifications for the warning, the child judges that disobedience will not get them into too much trouble, will not cause them any physical harm, and that, if they want to, they can stop

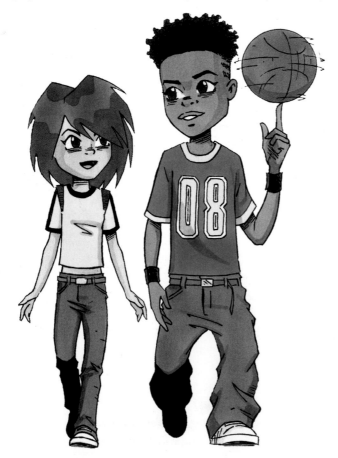

doing it. At this point, the child is effectively completely **IN CONTROL** of the level and duration of the act of **DISOBEYING**. In fact, children sometimes have to use willpower to ignore these warnings as they often don't especially want to use bad language, play with that friend or stay up late. Only rebelliousness prevents them from complying.

Warning category two:
'Don't do that because it will put you in danger.'
These are the warnings children are **LEAST** likely to ignore in order to **REBEL**. For example:

- *'Don't get in a car with a stranger.'*
- *'Don't cross the road without looking.'*
- *'Don't play with sharp objects.'*

Children may ignore these warnings at some stage, but rarely to spite their parents. They might forget the warning, not fully understand the importance of it in the first place, or be too embarrassed to heed it because of peer pressure. This is why, as parents, we try to highlight the warning by giving a valid reason for it – we identify a **REAL** danger:

- *'Don't get in a car with a stranger because they might do you harm.'*
- *'Don't cross the road without looking because you could be hit by a car.'*
- *'Don't play with sharp objects because you could cut yourself.'*

Children usually understand that the consequences of ignoring these warnings can be very serious and they don't often deliberately ignore them since that would not only get them in trouble with their parents but more importantly would risk hurting themselves **PHYSICALLY**, certainly **PAINFULLY** and possibly **FATALLY**. When such warnings are ignored it is usually accidental, because your child forgets the warning or doesn't realize the warning applies:

- *The child didn't get into the car with a stranger, it was a new friend.*
- *They weren't concentrating when they crossed the road.*
- *They didn't know it was so sharp.*

Parents can only give warnings in this category as effectively as possible in the hope that the child's instinct for survival will keep them safe.

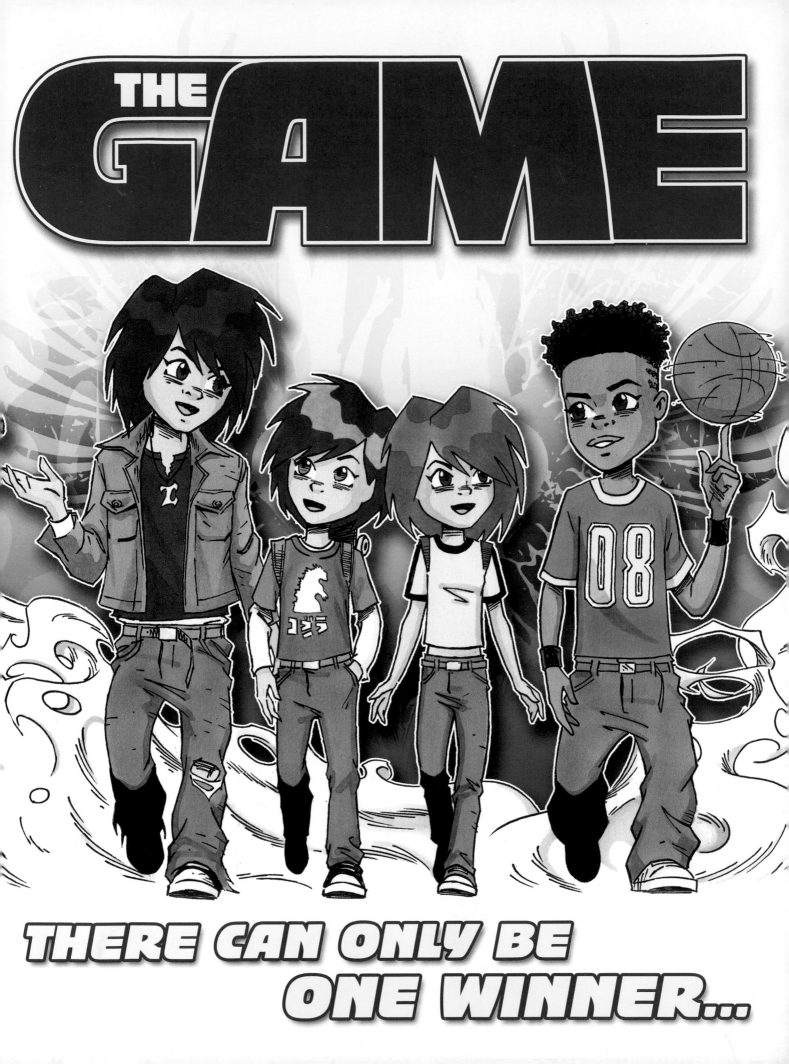

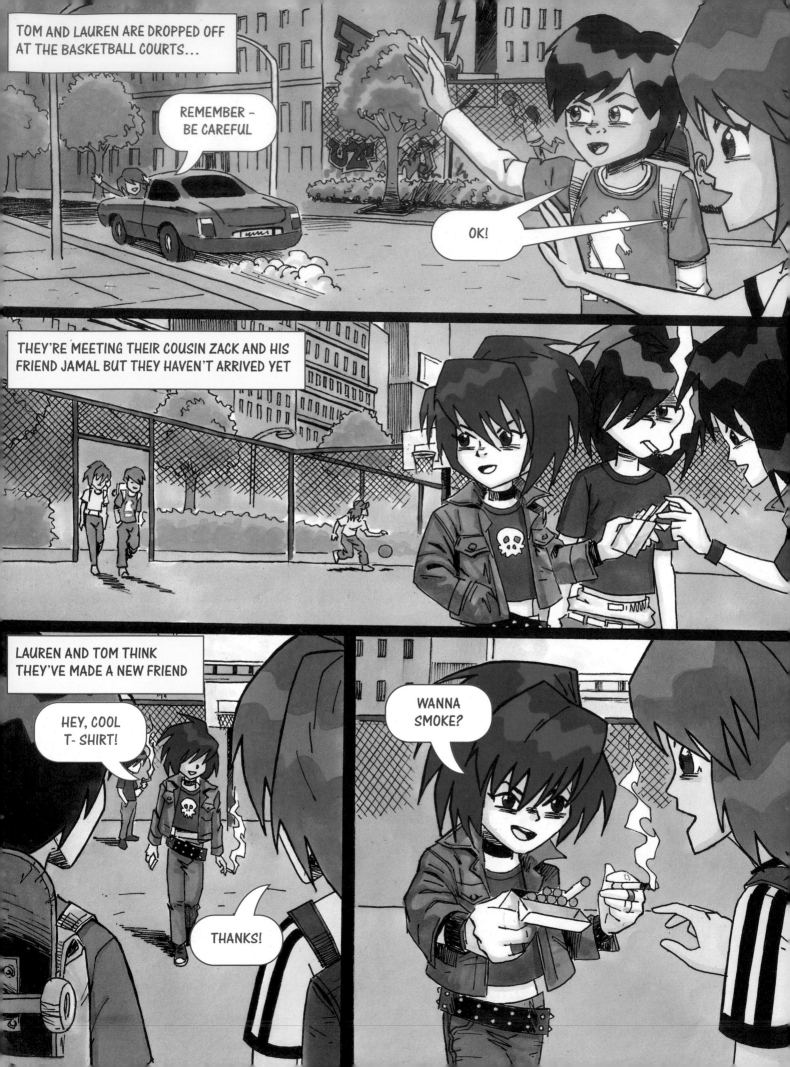

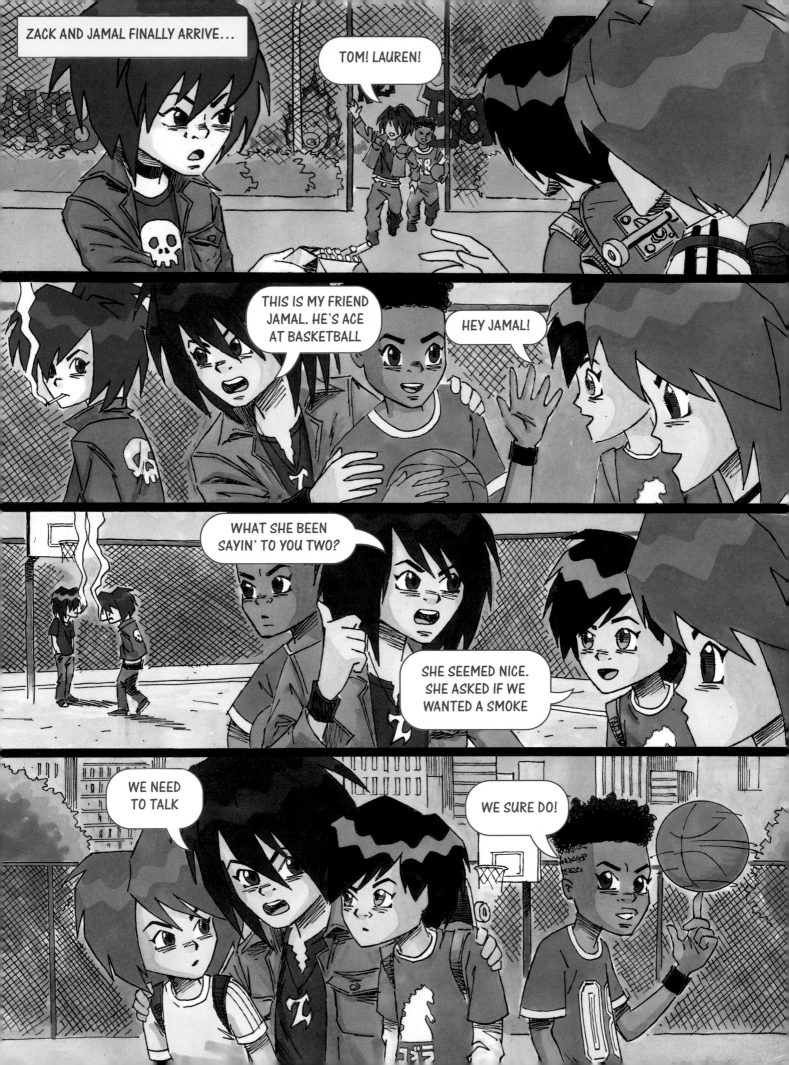

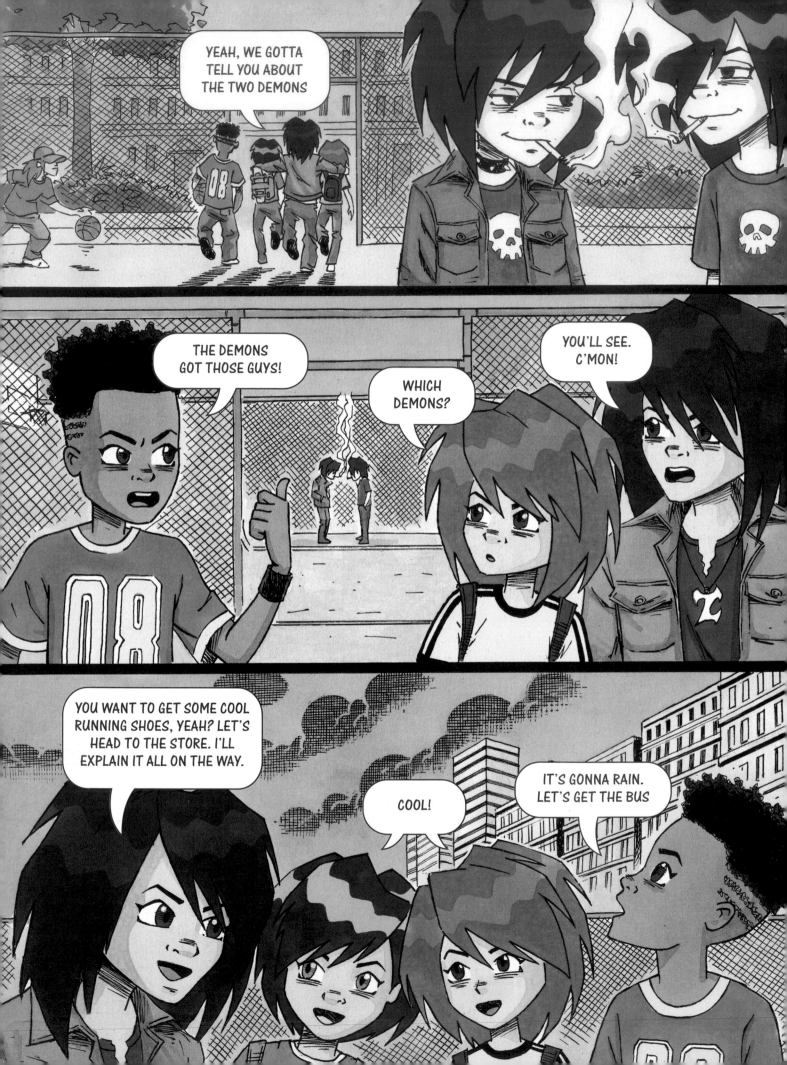

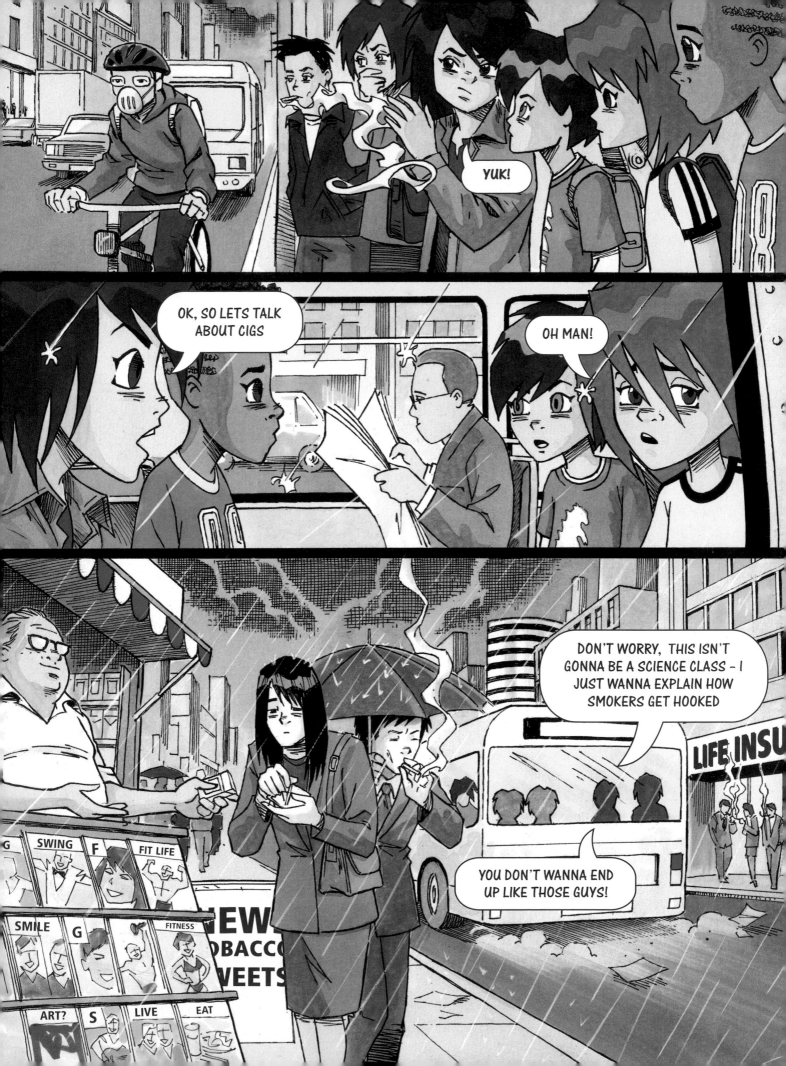

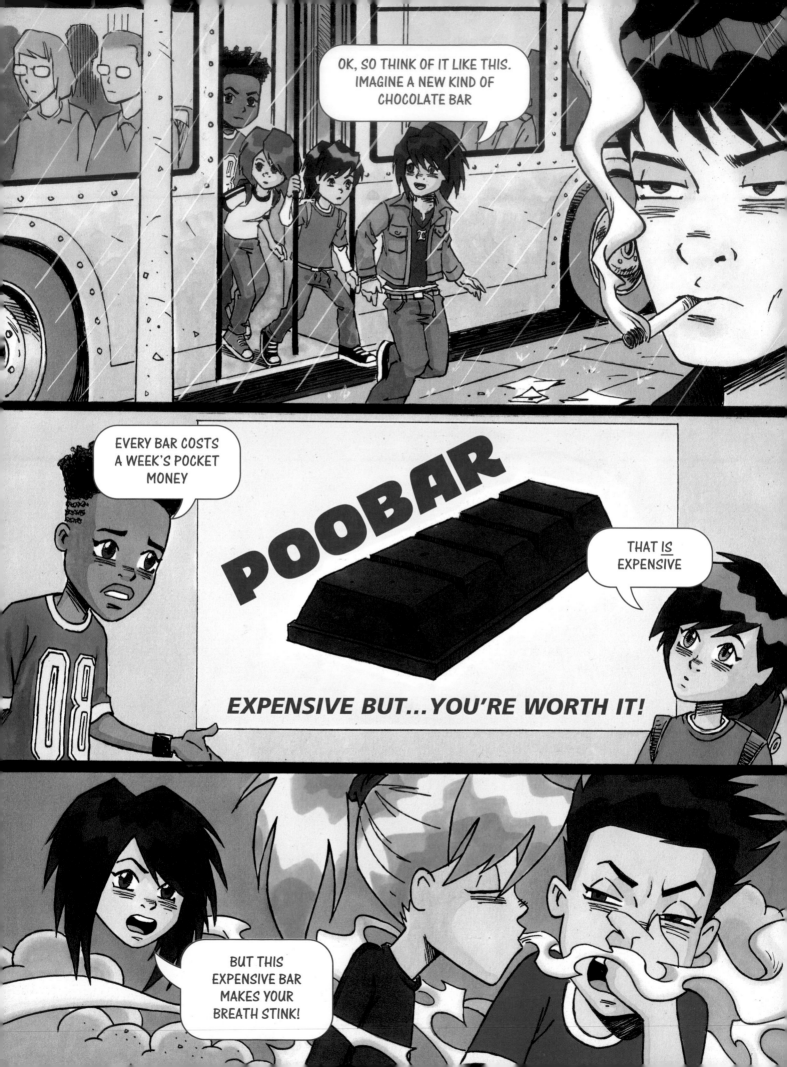

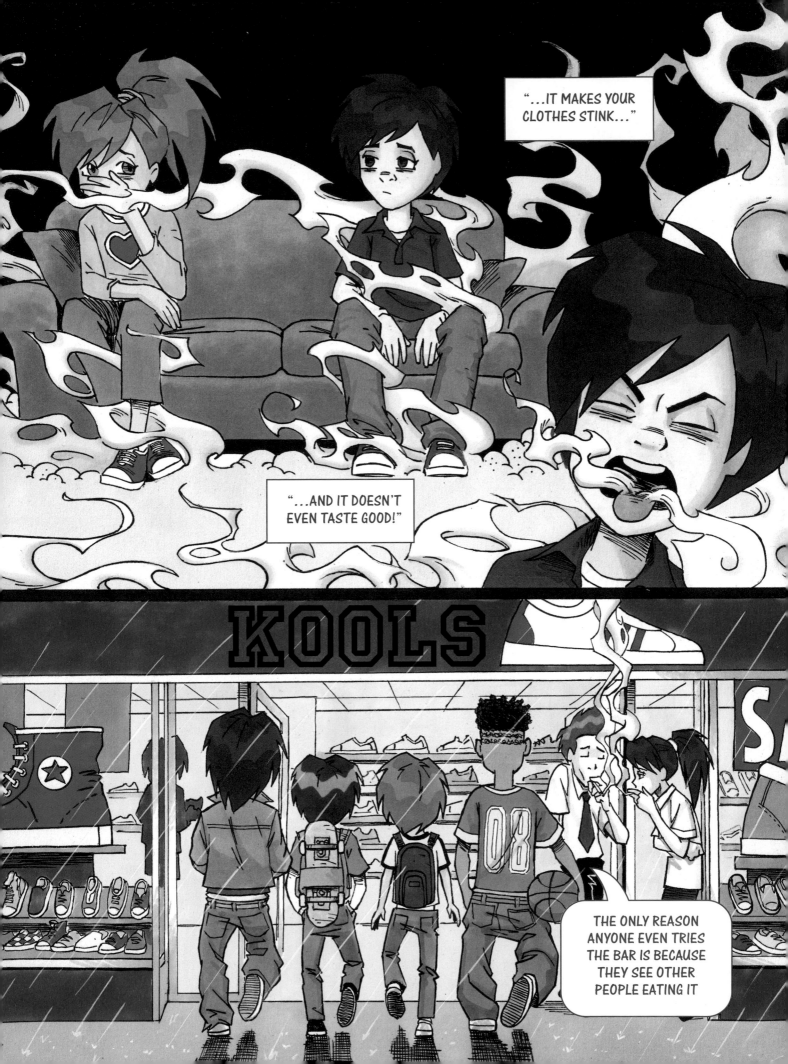

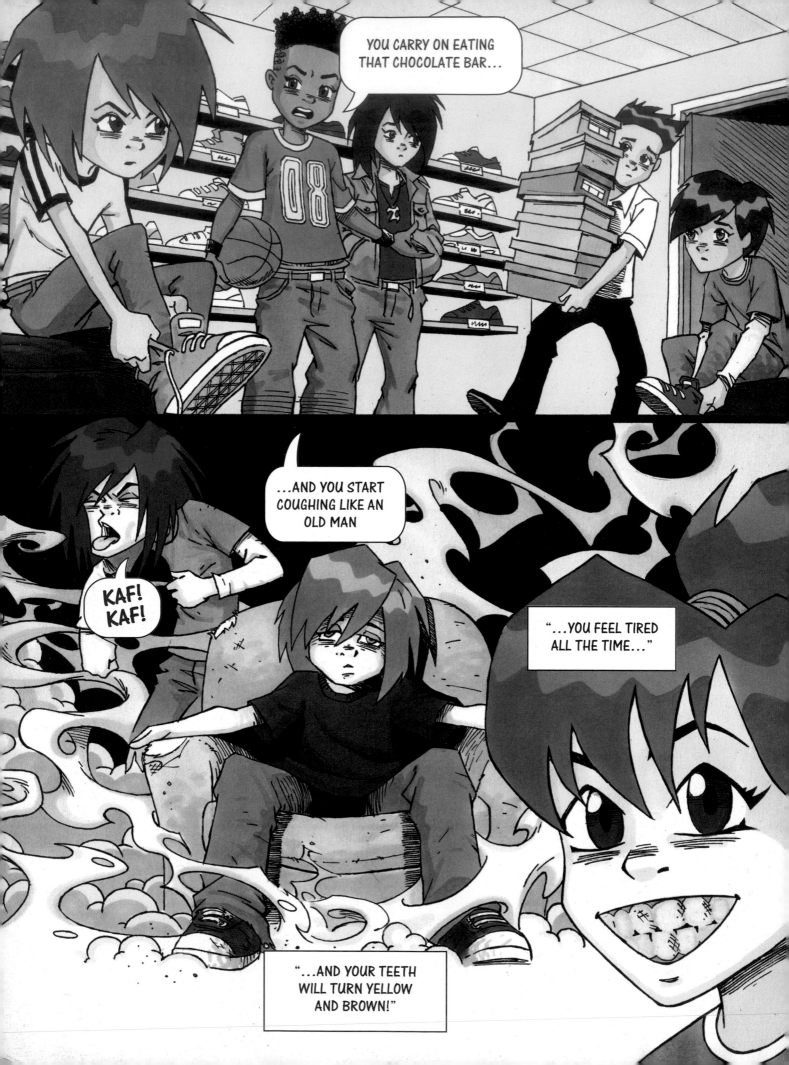

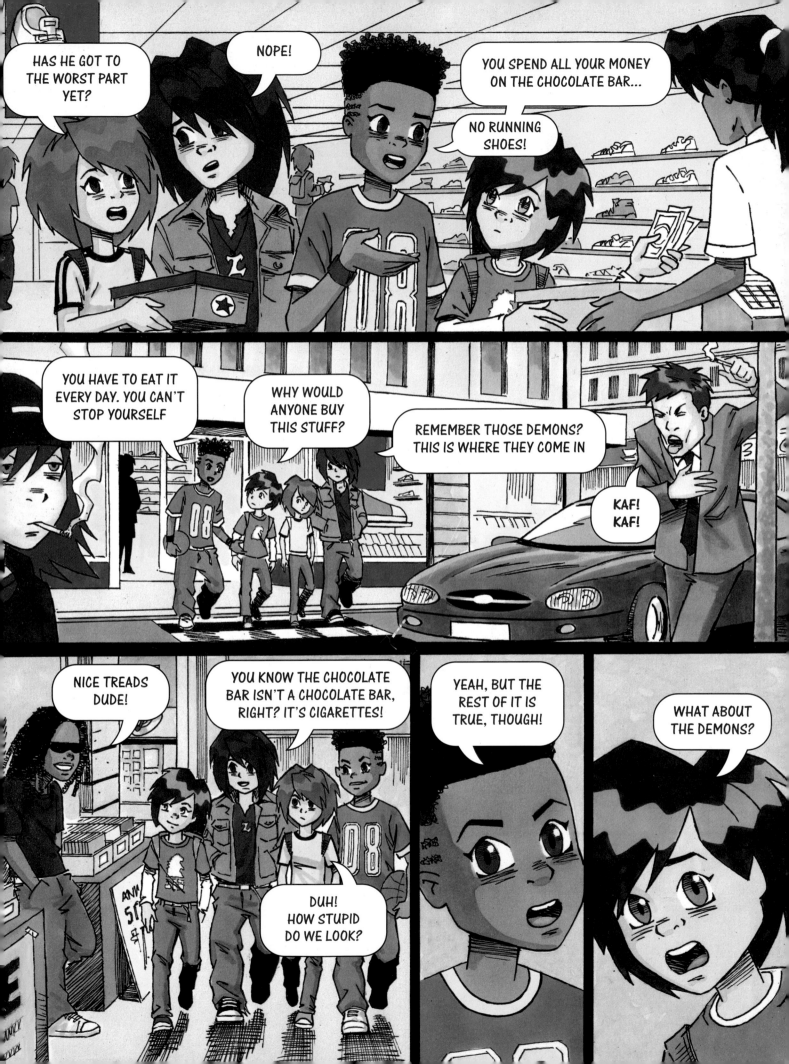

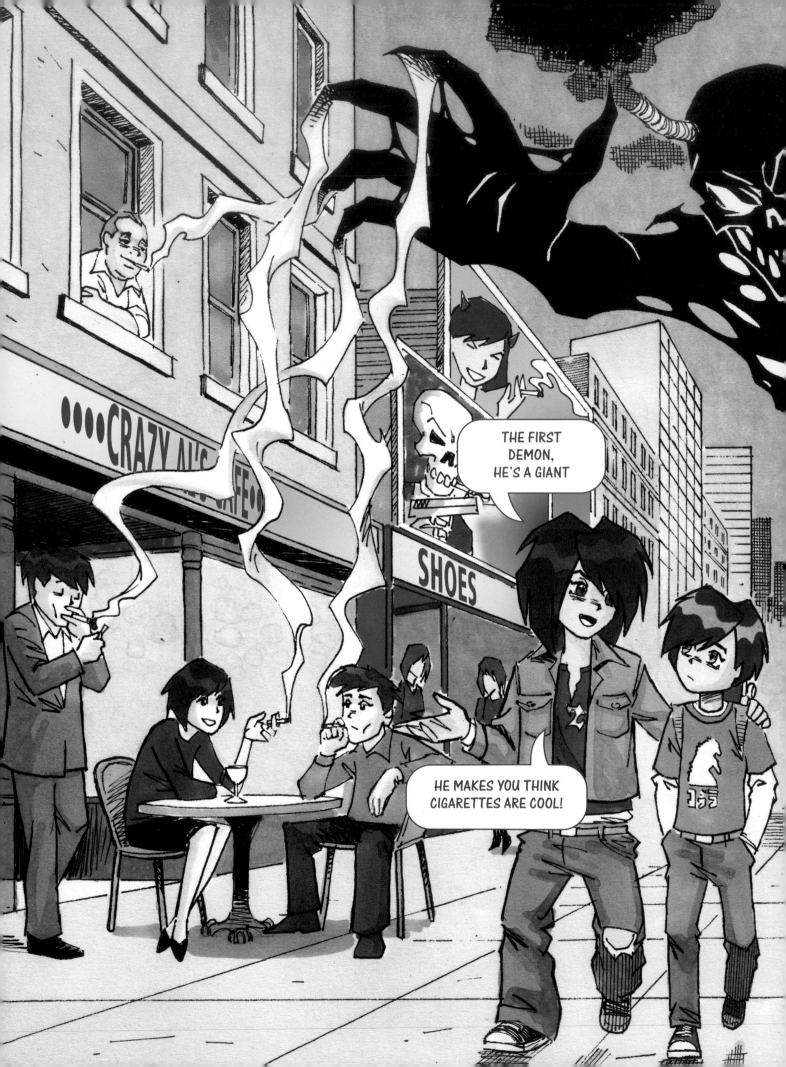

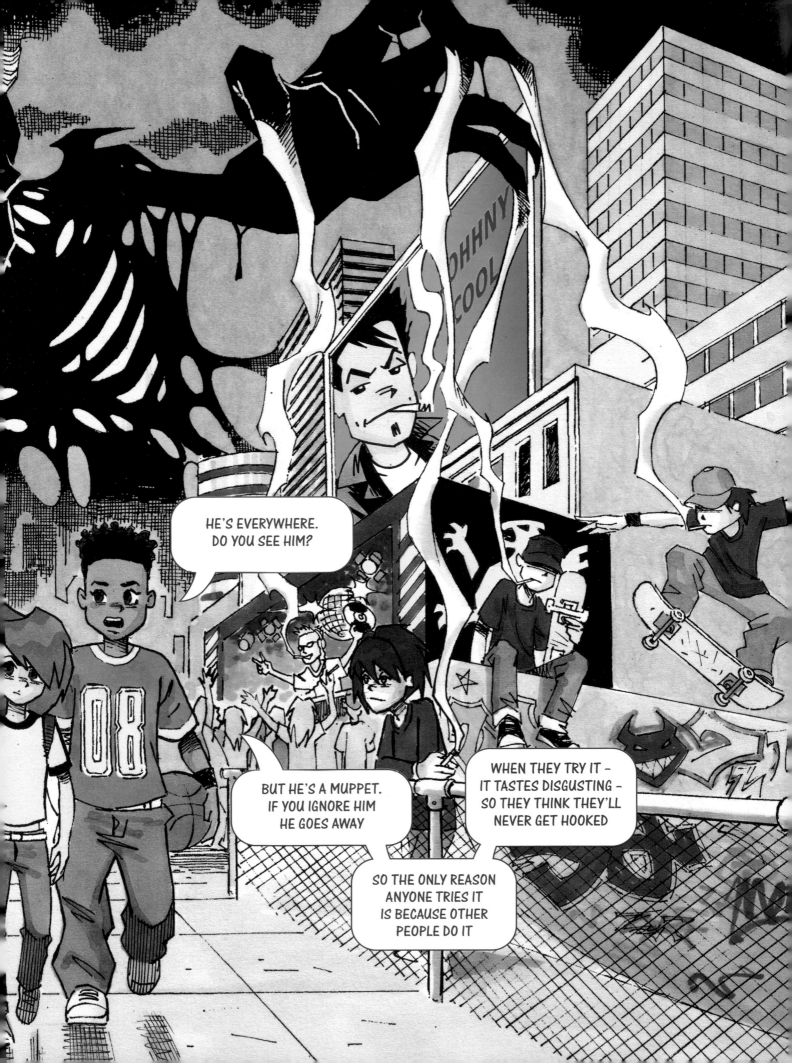

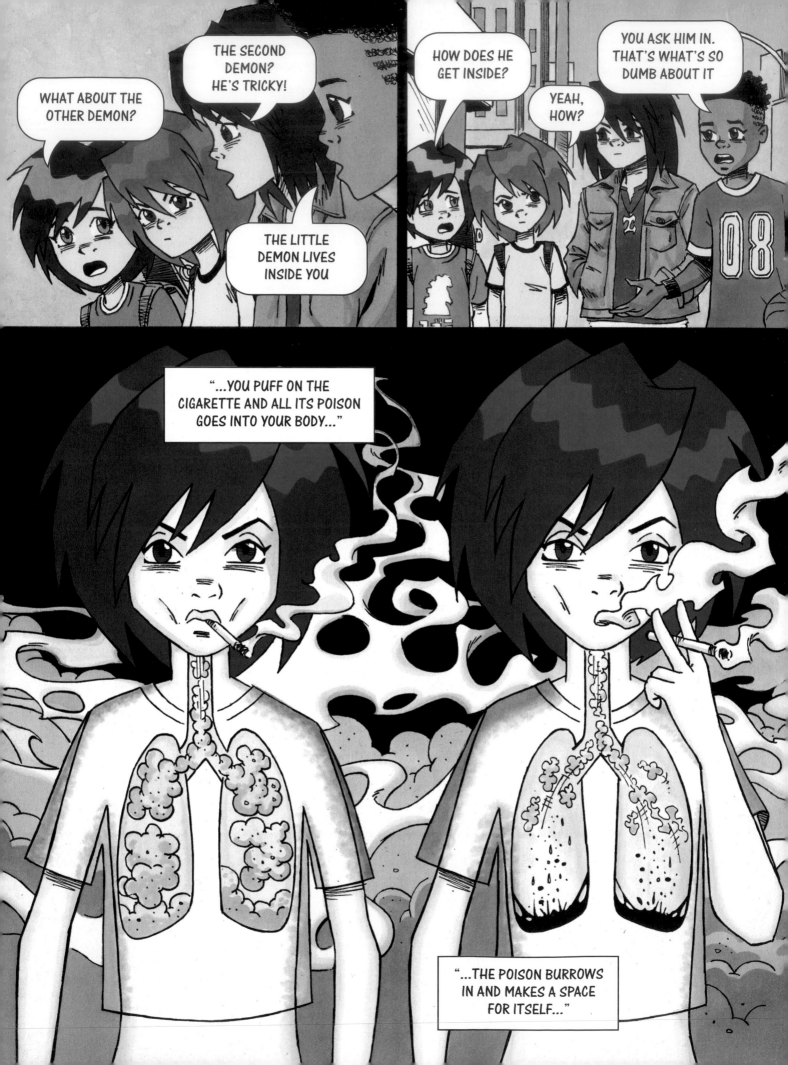

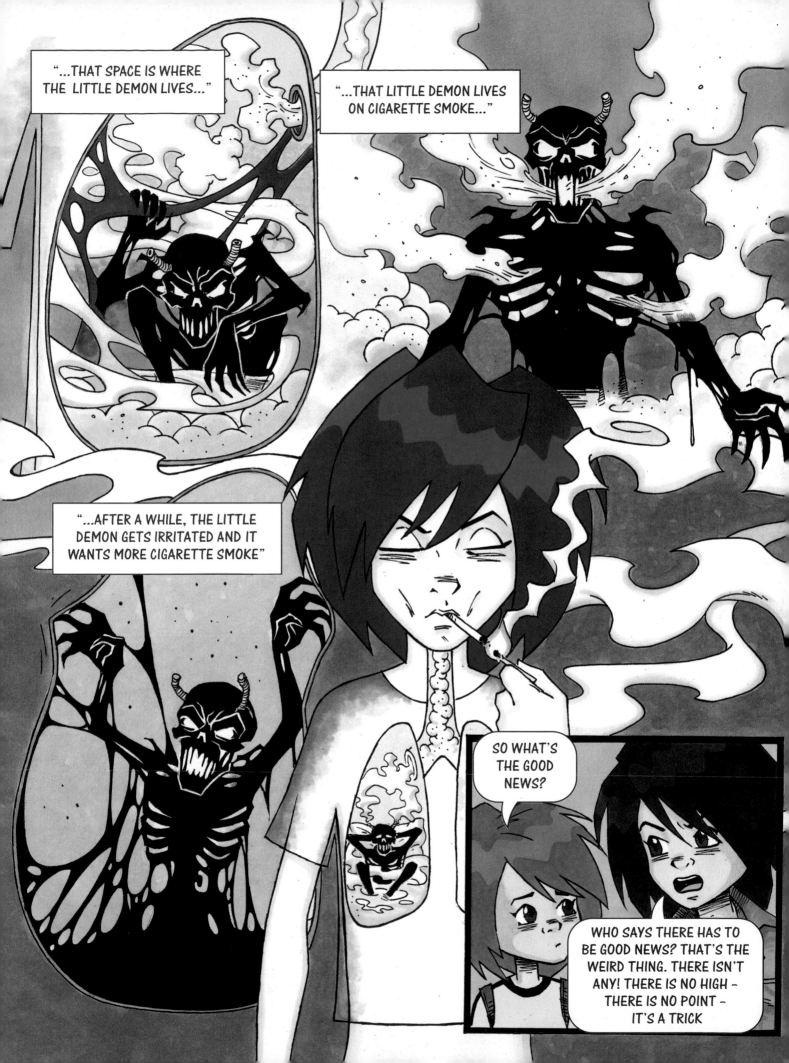

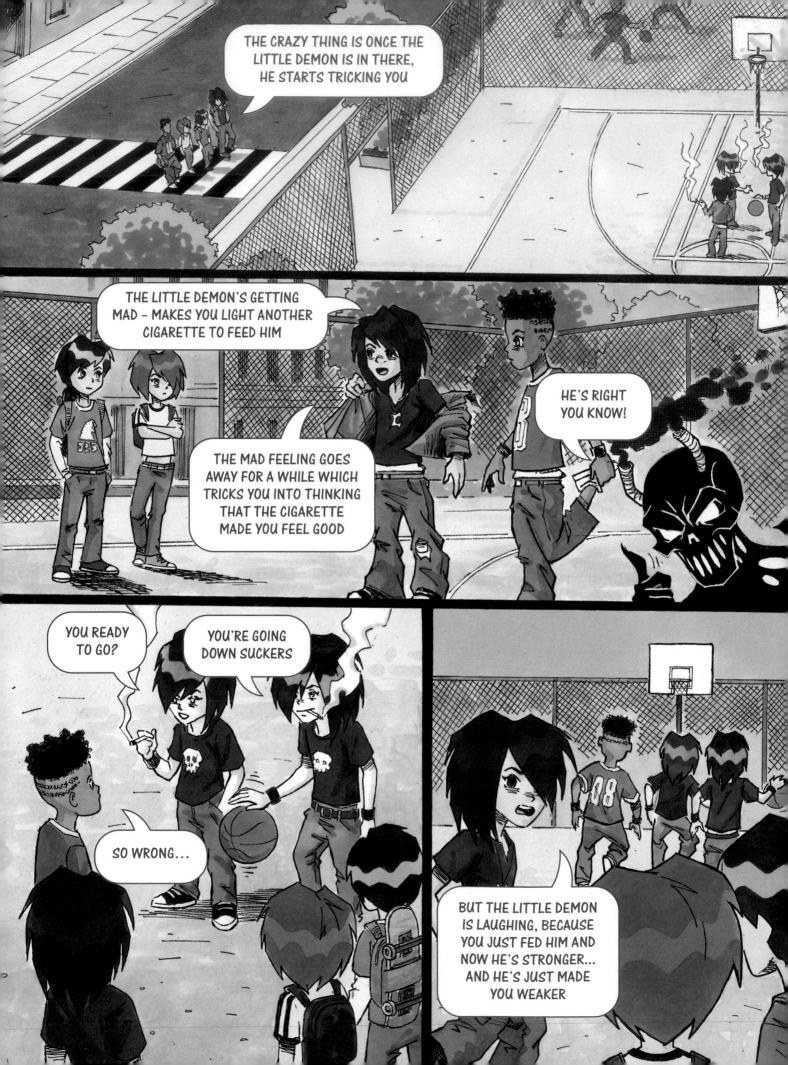

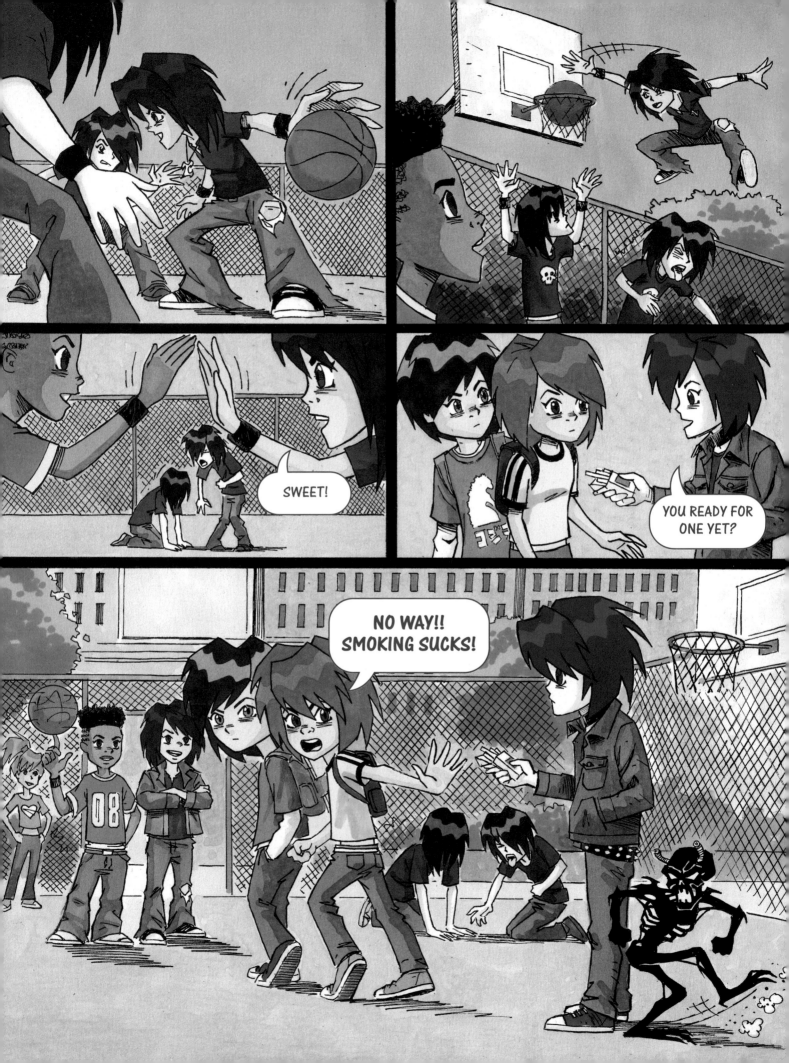

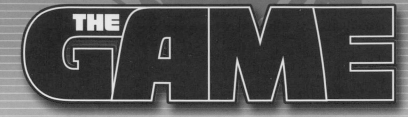

THE GAME

ON THE CITY BASKETBALL COURT, TENSIONS ARE RUNNING HIGH.
SMOKE IS RISING FROM THE TARMAC. THE DEMONS ARE WARMING UP
AND THE GAME IS ABOUT TO BEGIN. FRESH FROM THE COUNTRY,
SURELY UNDERDOGS TOM AND LAUREN DON'T STAND A CHANCE?

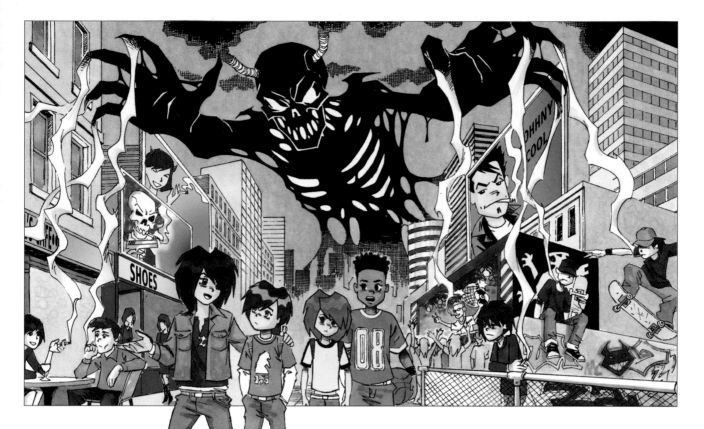

TACKLING SMOKING

Category one warnings

Many parents mistakenly apply category one warnings to smoking:

> *'Don't do it because I don't approve!'*

They often justify the warning by adding something like: 'It's stupid,' 'It stinks,' or 'You'll get hooked.' The child files this warning (along with their response to it) alongside the others that they receive in this category:

- *'Don't use bad language because it's rude!'* (Child thinks: *'I know it's rude, that's exactly WHY I do it!'*)
- *'Don't play with that friend because I don't like them.'* (Child thinks: *'I don't care if you don't like them, and anyway if it annoys you, so much the better!'*)
- *'Don't stay up late because you'll be tired in the morning!'* (Child thinks: *'So what? Going to bed early is for babies.'*)

REMEMBER – these are the warnings that the child is almost bound to dismiss and ignore (often deliberately).

Category two warnings

Many parents also apply category two warnings to smoking:

> *'Don't do it because it will put you in danger.'*

The problem is, they then justify their warning with an apparently phoney, inappropriate or ineffective explanation:

- *'Don't smoke because it will kill you.'* (Child thinks: *'No it won't. Auntie Jane, Uncle Jack and my teacher all smoke. They're not dead and they're REALLY old.'*)
- *'Don't smoke. Cigarettes killed your granddad.'* (Child thinks: *'OK, I don't really remember him much but he was ANCIENT!'*) Remember, it wouldn't matter if Granddad was only 50 when he died, as far as the child is concerned, he was virtually prehistoric!
- *'Don't smoke. Your dad wishes he never started.'* (Child thinks: *'GREAT! If it's all right for him, it's all right for me!! We go to football together, we go to the park together, one day we can smoke together! He's my hero. I want to be just like HIM, especially if it involves me getting away with being BAD!'*)

SO – WHAT CAN YOU DO?

Two things will help you stop your child taking up smoking: creating a non-smoking environment, and education about smoking.

Start early

MINIMIZE the extent to which your child is exposed to smoking both physically and visually. Apart from the health effects of passive smoking, do you really want your child to grow up thinking that smoking is normal, acceptable behaviour? Your attitude should be that family and friends are welcome to smoke wherever they want *EXCEPT* near or in view of your child. You won't be able to eliminate your child's exposure completely – they'll see smokers on the street and on TV – but *YOU* should take responsibility for controlling your relatives and friends.

If you smoke

If you smoke yourself, take this opportunity to stop now. Don't kid yourself that you will be able to hide it from your children – *YOU WON'T!* They identify the *SMELL* of their parents. Do you want them to identify you with the stench of stale cigarettes? If your children know you are smoking, any warnings, guidance, advice or education you give will have *ZERO* credibility. If you don't want your children to smoke, that means you wish you didn't smoke yourself. Allen Carr's Easyway enables you to stop easily, painlessly and permanently by removing the need and desire to smoke. It removes the fear of stopping and the feeling of deprivation. You'll enjoy social occasions more and handle stress better the moment you *GET FREE*. Most important of all, *YOU WON'T MISS CIGARETTES*. So quit now for the purely selfish reason that you'll enjoy life so much more as a non-smoker and then you'll also reap the reward of being able to help your children avoid the trap. For details of Allen Carr's Easyway books and clinics see the end of this booklet, or visit **www.allencarr.com**

If you are an ex-smoker

If you used to smoke yourself, tell your child that starting was one of the biggest mistakes you ever made; that you never thought that you would get hooked just by smoking a few cigarettes; that you spent XXXX thousand pounds on it and got nothing in return (the calculation is £5 multiplied by the number of packs you smoked per day, multiplied by the number of days you smoked. For a 20-a-day smoker who smokes for 20 years, that's £36,500); that

although you hated it, you felt you couldn't stop until you did manage to quit; and that stopping was one of the best things you've ever done.

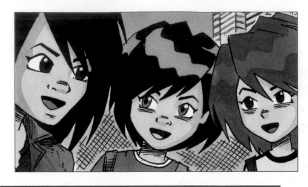

HOW THE COMIC WORKS

In the same way that responsible parents take time to explain the facts of life to their children, you need to take time and care to explain the facts about smoking as well. This booklet will help you understand and explain to your children *THE FACTS ABOUT SMOKING* and how to *AVOID THE SMOKING TRAP*. The comic has been written by experts who understand what makes children start smoking. It has been carefully designed to address these issues in a way that appeals to children during the age groups when they are most likely to fall into the trap. The comic strip deals with the following issues in ways children can relate to:

- *How peer pressure can make it hard to say no to cigarettes;*
- *How marketing from the tobacco industry bombards children with images of 'cool' smokers;*
- *Some of the health effects of smoking: these are outlined in the text and shown in the illustrations of the characters;*
- *How cigarette addiction happens, and how it seems difficult to 'unhook' yourself once the cigarette demon has got inside you;*
- *The negative social effects of smoking, such as how your clothes and breath stink.*

Our research shows that the colourful manga-style characters in the comic appeal to children. The visual elements in the comic allow them to pick up on the non-smoking messages without feeling patronized. The characters also use the everyday language of young people. This prevents them from feeling that they are reading a school textbook or other instructive material giving category one or two warnings.

The age of your child and his or her reading ability will determine how best to use this comic and get the message across most successfully. Your child can find out more about the main characters in the story as well as quizzes and games at **www.smokingsucks.co.uk**

Younger children

For younger children, it is best to read through the comic with them at a quiet time. By introducing the comic as something new and fun to read, your child will be interested in the story and the characters. At various points in the story you can stop and ask them questions, such as what they think is going to happen and who they think looks 'cool'. By asking your child's views about the characters in the comic, you can make them feel more involved. After finishing, you can discuss what they think about smoking and ask them if they think smoking is a good idea. By asking their opinion, they feel that they are being treated as individuals and in control of their own decisions.

Older children

For older children who are at the age when they may be thinking of starting smoking, or have already started, you can leave them to read the comic by themselves. You can give the comic to them, suggesting that they have a look and tell you what they think of it. If your child becomes defensive when you raise the subject of smoking, or you feel that they would not respond well, you can take a different approach. Just leave the comic in their bedroom, by the front door or in the bathroom. This way, they can pick it up when they feel ready to read it, in their own time. Encourage your children to take the comic to school to share with their peers. It will serve as a powerful tool to help them resist peer pressure at school, where smoking is often seen as cool. When faced with the suggestion of smoking, they have a 'support' in the form of a cool comic.

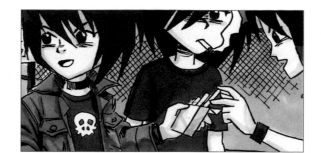

FINAL NOTE

Remember, at some point your child will almost certainly be offered a cigarette. You will almost certainly not be there, and your child will have to make a decision by himself/herself. Education is the best way you can help your child to make the right decision. And no one can doubt that, where smoking is concerned, **PREVENTION** is better than **CURE**.

Smoking Sucks! cannot guarantee to prevent your children from starting smoking but it can weigh the odds as heavily in their favour as possible. Follow our advice, prevent the next generation of smokers from even starting, and help us fulfil Allen Carr's goal: to cure the world of smoking.

ALLEN CARR'S EASYWAY CLINICS

Below are the contact details for all Allen Carr Stop Smoking Clinics worldwide where the success rate, based on the money-back guarantee, is over 90%. Selected clinics also offer sessions dealing with alcohol and weight issues. Please check with your nearest clinic for details. Find out where it is from the address opposite. Allen Carr guarantees you will find it easy to stop smoking at his clinics or your money back. Allen Carr's Easyway Clinics operate in more than 35 countries worldwide.

www.allencarr.com

Allen Carr's Easyway – Worldwide Head Office

Park House, 14 Pepys Road, Raynes Park,
London SW20 8NH
Tel: **+44 (0)208 9447761**
Email: **mail@allencarr.com**
Website: **www.allencarr.com**

Worldwide Press Office

Tel: **+44 (0)7970 88 44 52**
Email: **jd@statacom.net**

UK Clinic Information and Central Booking Line:
0800 389 2115 (*Freephone*)

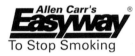

Allen Carr's
Easyway ®
To Stop Smoking

Allen Carr's
SMOKING SUCKS!
HELP YOUR CHILDREN AVOID THE SMOKING TRAP

Written by Allen Carr and Robin Hayley
Comic written in conjunction with Paul Mason
Illustrator: Steve Beaumont
Editor: Fiona Tulloch
Designers: Steve Flight and Peter Ridley

To our children, grandchildren and great grandchildren
*– **Allen Carr and Robin Hayley***

ARCTURUS

Arcturus Publishing Limited
26/27 Bickels Yard
151–153 Bermondsey Street
London SE1 3HA

Published in association with
foulsham
W. Foulsham & Co. Ltd,
The Publishing House, Bennetts Close, Cippenham,
Slough, Berkshire SL1 5AP, England

ISBN: 978-0-572-03320-0

British Library Cataloguing-in-Publication Data: a catalogue record for this book is available from the British Library

This edition printed in 2007

Text copyright © 2007 Allen Carr's Easyway (International) Limited
Design copyright © 2007 Arcturus Publishing Limited

Printed in Malaysia

--- **SPECIAL NOTE** ---

The world's leading expert on stopping smoking, Allen Carr, was diagnosed with lung cancer in the summer of 2006. He passed away peacefully in his sleep on 29th November 2006 with his wife, Joyce, at his bedside. Allen's illness was thought to have been caused by the years he spent in smoke-filled rooms, treating smokers at his clinics. When asked if cancer was too high a cost, his reply was always the same: 'When I stubbed out my last cigarette 23 years ago I became the happiest man in the world – I still feel the same way today. I've been told that my books and clinics have cured more than 10 million smokers, in which case I think it is a price worth paying.'